Table of content

Chapter 1

Building Physical Vitality Across The Lifespan

Introduction

Physical vitality is essential for living life to the fullest across all life stages. It provides the energy, strength, mobility and resilience to fulfill our roles, pursue goals, and enjoy everyday activities free of exhaustion or limitation. Physical vitality enhances mental health, disease resistance, self-confidence, and quality of life while enabling greater productivity and longevity. This chapter will define physical vitality and outline how it can be cultivated through proper nutrition, adequate fitness, quality sleep, health-conscious habits, preventative care, and adapting routines as we age. Specific strategies will be tailored to each phase - childhood, adolescence, early adulthood, middle age, and senior years. A lifetime approach is key, as good health results from the compound benefits of continuous healthy routines sustained consistently over decades. With diligent yet balanced attention to our changing physical needs as we grow older, we can maintain vibrancy, independence and engagement with life.

Childhood

In childhood, vitality comes naturally through abundant energy expended freely through active play, curiosity, and a desire to explore life. Maximizing physical development and fitness from an early age establishes positive lifelong health trajectories. According to physical activity guidelines, toddlers and preschoolers should engage in at least 3 hours of energetic active play daily with both structured and unstructured activities. Physical education classes, outdoor free play, organized sports, and family exercises like hiking or biking help young children build cardiovascular endurance, motor skills, movement confidence, and healthy habits. Aerobic, muscle-strengthening, and bone-strengthening activities are all beneficial. Adequate nutrition provides the fuel and building blocks for growth and development. Pediatricians recommend limited screen time, 10+ hours of quality sleep nightly, safety measures like bike helmets, and age-appropriate immunizations and well-child checkups to monitor development. Instilling healthy routines and protections early on benefits children lifelong.

Adolescence

As children enter adolescence, adequate nutrition and exercise become even more critical to support pubertal changes and fuel rapid growth. Teens have increased caloric needs balanced with ample proteins, vitamins, minerals, calcium for bone mass, and iron for menstruating girls. Physical activity guidelines recommend at least 1 hour of moderate to vigorous activity daily combining aerobic exercise, muscle training, and bone-strengthening activities. Sports participation provides fitness along with social and teamwork skills. Strength training with free weights develops lean muscle mass. Stretching maintains flexibility. Yet teens must avoid overexercising or excessive attempts at bodily perfection. Sleep habits degrade when nightly sleep needs remain around 9 hours. Good sleep hygiene helps teens arrive at school alert and supports mood regulation. Pediatricians track growth and development markers while providing guidance on needed immunizations, sexual health, hygiene, and avoidance of risky behaviors like drug use or reckless driving. Ongoing medical care and open communication keeps adolescents healthy.

Early Adulthood

As young adults transition into college, career, and independent living, many experience declining fitness and nutrition. Without athletic teams or family meals, young professionals often cope with long work hours and stress through convenience eating, screen overuse, social drinking, and lack of exercise. However, timesaving strategies like food prep on weekends, gym sessions before work, joining fitness classes or recreational leagues, and taking breaks from desk jobs can sustain vitality. Healthy relationships providing camaraderie, purpose and work-life balance protect against burnout. As metabolism naturally slows with age, maintaining healthy weight requires reducing calories along with regular physical activity and strength training. Young adults may feel invulnerable but should continue recommended screenings, dental visits, and immunizations while minimizing exposure to infections through safe hygiene and sexual habits. Building lifelong positive habits now prevents disease and decline later.

Middle Adulthood

By midlife, health consciousness becomes critical as metabolism continues slowing, risk factors like obesity and hypertension rise, and chronic conditions manifest. However, concerted efforts can minimize typical declines. Daily moderate activity sustained over decades provides cardiovascular, muscular, and mental health benefits. Adults should perform muscle-strengthening activities at least twice weekly and balance challenges for fall prevention. Stretching maintains joint flexibility too. Adapting long-loved sports to prevent overuse injuries enables continuance. Nutrition should shift to anti-inflammatory foods like produce, whole grains, and healthy fats while restricting sugar, salt and cholesterol. Adequate protein intake is important to preserve lean muscle mass. Quality sleep may require improved sleep hygiene. Annual physicals allow early screening, intervention, and monitoring while immunizations protect against viruses still posing threats like influenza, pneumonia and shingles. Midlife vitality requires heightened intention, adaptation and prevention.

Later Adulthood

Seniors face declining strength, mobility, stamina, and physiological resilience but remaining active with appropriate modifications allows many to preserve capable vitality into later decades. Light cardiovascular and strengthening exercises improve balance, mobility and mood while reducing risks of falls and disability. Stretching maintains joint flexibility and function. Walking, swimming and water workouts provide gentle activity options. Movement limitations can be adapted with chair exercises, resistance bands, or home routines with grab bars and stability assistance. Understandable frustration with activity reductions should be countered by focusing on continuing lifelong hobbies adapted to current abilities. Later adulthood requires extra attention to bone health through sufficient calcium and vitamin D. Social engagement provides both emotional fulfillment and motivation for activity. Cognitive health should be protected through ongoing learning and games. Annual wellness visits allow coordination of care between providers to manage chronic conditions optimally. Proactively addressing changing health needs helps sustain vitality and independence.

Conclusion

Our physical health evolves across our lifespans, influenced by genetics, nutrition, fitness, stress levels and environmental exposures. Certain factors remain within our control. A lifetime approach focused on optimal wellbeing starting early and adapting appropriately as we age provides the best opportunity for avoiding preventable ill health and decline associated with a sedentary modern lifestyle. Childhood is the best time to instill healthy nutrition, activity enjoyment, and safety habits that will carry forward into adulthood. Teens should be guided to balance adolescent urges and self-consciousness with reasonable fitness and self-care routines. Adulthood requires prioritizing our health amidst busy careers and families through meal planning, stress management techniques and consistent exercise. Midlife is the time for targeted disease prevention and adapting existing routines to changing capabilities. Seniors must proactively address evolving limited mobility and strength through light, balanced fitness regimens utilizing appropriate modifications. While each life stage has unique considerations, sustaining daily movement, healthy diets, medical prevention, restorative sleep, and social connections will provide benefits across the decades. With intention and self-compassion, we can take charge of our evolving physical vitality and health needs to thrive through all of life's seasons from childhood to eventually centenarian status and beyond.

Chapter 2

Maintaining Brain Health And Cognitive Vitality Across The Lifespan

The human brain is remarkably malleable, with the ability to create new neural connections and adapt in response to stimulation. While some cognitive decline is inevitable with aging, sustaining brain health maximizes functioning. This chapter will explain brain development changes across life stages, factors influencing cognition, and science-based strategies tailored to different age groups to maintain mental acuity. Just as physical exercise strengthens the body, regular brain exercise builds cognitive reserve. Combining learning, skill-building, socializing and healthy lifestyles provides benefits across the decades.

Brain Development Overview

In utero, neurons rapidly proliferate, then prune for efficiency. Infancy and childhood see dramatic brain growth and neural wiring. The hippocampus manages memory while the prefrontal cortex handles executive functions. During adolescence, gray matter thins and neural connections refine. Early adulthood is the cognitive peak. After age 20, certain skills like processing speed slowly decline while crystallized abilities like vocabulary remain stable. From midlife on, some short-term memory loss is expected along with slower recall. However, neuroplasticity allows learning at any age by forming new connections. Novel challenges create fresh neural networks while repetitive tasks reinforce existing ones. Education, occupations, lifestyle habits and genetics also shape cognition over decades. With intention, we can minimize expected losses.

Assessing Cognition Across Life Stages

Standardized tests like IQ assessments measure abilities like memory, attention, processing speed and problem-solving.

School achievement tests evaluate skills like reading, writing and math. Neuropsychological testing diagnoses impairments through targeted cognitive tasks. Brain imaging visualizes structure and activity differences. For children, development milestones reflect emerging abilities - walking, talking, reading etc. Schools administer achievement tests periodically. For adults, mental status exams test orientation, recall, language use and attention. Executive functioning tests measure planning and cognitive flexibility. Normal cognitive changes due to aging must be distinguished from pathological deterioration suggesting disorders like dementia. Tracking cognitive performance over time personalizes expected trajectories. Self-monitoring mental functioning also helps identify needs.

Strategies to Strengthen Cognition
Cognition depends on brain health supported through stimulation, nutrition, socializing, exercise and stress management. Each life stage has tailored needs. Young children require interactive play, varied environments, language engagement and rest. School-age enrichment includes reading, hobbies, arts, sports and socializing. Teens benefit from intellectual challenges, youth groups and teaching resilience. Higher education and mentoring develop adult cognition. Learning new skills and occupational demands challenge working adults. Midlife requires learning coping strategies while health factors are proactively managed. Seniors should stay active socially and intellectually with games, classes and volunteering. Mixed exercise, memory exercises and healthy diets nourish brains lifelong. Train the brain like a muscle with increasingly complex tasks. But balance challenges with recovery. Believing in your own potential matters too.

Activities That Strengthen Cognition
Physical activity, games, creative arts, socializing, higher education and engaging careers provide cognitive benefits. Aerobic exercise improves focus while dance integrates

physical and cognitive skills. Exercising the mind directly through increasingly difficult puzzles, logic problems or strategy games builds mental stamina. Reading fiction fosters imagination and empathy. Learning musical instruments sharpens auditory, motor and memory regions simultaneously. Performing arts integrate physical, emotional and intellectual abilities. Writing improves linguistic skills, organization and creativity. Photography and other visual arts strengthen visual processing and spatial awareness. Travel and exposure to diverse cultures and perspectives prevent insular thinking. Higher education develops critical analysis and specialization. Mentally demanding careers involving complex decision-making bolster cognitive reserves. Social involvement provides stimulation while a sense of purpose may protect against cognitive decline.

Strengthening Cognition Through Lifestyle Factors
Optimal nutrition supports every body system, including the brain. The Mediterranean diet rich in produce, lean proteins, nuts and healthy fats provides antioxidants, B vitamins, and anti-inflammatory benefits. Restful sleep clears neuronal waste while consolidating memory and learning. Emotional support and close relationships prevent isolation while providing meaning. Stress management preserves plasticity and new learning. Certain supplements like fish oil may aid memory but require medical guidance. Engaging hobbies, arts, games and community service give a sense of fulfillment. Remain open to learning new things, meeting new people, traveling and discovering possibilities. Protect hearing and vision to avoid sensory deprivation. Manage conditions like obesity, hypertension, high cholesterol and diabetes that heighten dementia risk. With comprehensive lifestyle attention, cognitive declines can be minimized.

Inspiring Examples of Lifelong Learners

Many high achievers remain intellectually engaged into older age by sustaining curiosity, embracing learning and contributing their wisdom. Examples include: Warren Buffet still directing investments in his 90s; Tony Bennett singing into his 90s; Noam Chomsky writing books in his 90s; Supreme Court Justice Ruth Ginsberg serving into her 80s; Clint Eastwood directing films in his 80s; Nancy Pelosi remaining House Speaker in her 80s; Jane Goodall still doing chimpanzee research in her 80s; Ed Whitlock set running records into his 80s; Maya Angelou had a prolific writing career into her 80s; Betty White acted into her 90s; Queen Elizabeth II still performing duties in her 90s; Roger Waters touring in his 70s; Suzanne Somers acting in her 70s; Martha Stewart active in business in her 70s. Leaders prove that with intention, much can be accomplished in later decades.

Conclusion

Our brains remain malleable for learning and compensation across our lifespans when continuously stimulated. Some loss is inevitable but engaging interests, activities and communities can counteract declines. Each life phase has cognitive needs - toddlers need discovery of their world, teens need identity development, adults need career building and mentors, seniors need intellectual community. Good nutrition, exercise and sleep support optimal functioning. By believing in our potential and embracing lifelong learning habits, we can live meaningfully at every age. As the saying goes "use it or lose it" - keeping brains active reduces the risk of neurological diseases later on. Modern science continues making advances in understanding how to optimize brain health. But individually, we can support our cognition across decades through lifestyle choices that exercise, nourish and protect our minds. With intention, intellectual curiosity endures while wisdom accrues.

Chapter 3

building emotional resilience and mental wellbeing across the lifespan

Our emotional health evolves across our lives as we encounter varied stressors, experiences, and changes. Some anguish and frustration is inevitable but we can mitigate negative impacts by developing emotional resilience. This chapter will explain mental health changes across life stages, factors influencing resilience, and science-based strategies tailored to different age groups to sustain emotional wellbeing. Just as we strengthen our bodies through fitness, we can condition our minds to handle adversities through building coping skills, social support networks, and therapeutic outlets. With intention, we can become more emotionally agile and resilient at any age.

Emotional Development Overview

In infancy, developing secure caregiver attachments and trust provide an emotional foundation. The limbic system, which governs emotion, emerges early. As language skills progress, identifying and communicating feelings becomes possible. During childhood, play enables processing experiences and practicing social skills. Self-awareness and regulation improves with maturity of the prefrontal cortex. Adolescence brings heightened emotions, self-consciousness, risk-taking, and susceptibility to peer influences. Early adulthood requires independence and self-reliance. Relationships take on more significance. Middle age may be stressful balancing competing priorities and responsibilities. Fear of aging escalates with physical declines. Senior years require emotional adaptation to loss of loved ones, limitations and life reflection. Emotional wisdom often emerges from lifelong experiences. Personality, coping abilities, mental health and cognitive fitness all affect emotional health over decades.

Assessing Mental Wellbeing

Standardized assessments like depression and anxiety inventories screen for common conditions using symptom scales. Resilience assessments measure optimism, flexibility, coping and self-efficacy through questionnaires. Emotional intelligence tests evaluate abilities like self-awareness, self-regulation, empathy and motivation. Developmental milestones reflect emerging social-emotional skills. Academic and behavioral performance can indicate distresses. Adults self-report life satisfaction, positive moods and purpose. For seniors, geriatric depression scales identify issues needing intervention. Tracking mental health data over time personalizes expected baselines. Journaling, completing positive psychology exercises and discussing feelings with supportive connections also provide insights. Therapy helps overcome traumas and destructive thought patterns through tools like Cognitive Behavioral approaches. As with physical fitness, regularly assessing and working to improve mental fitness is beneficial.

Strategies to Strengthen Mental Resilience

Developing resilient emotional health requires nurturing supportive relationships, productive outlets for stress, therapeutic care when needed, coping strategies tailored to life stage and priorities, balancing obligations with self-care, limiting behaviors that provide only illusory relief like overeating or drugs, maintaining a sense of purpose, creativity and humor, practicing gratitude and living in the present. Positive emotions actually build resilience by quieting fear centers and fueling motivation. Challenging yet achievable goals provide a sense of accomplishment. Reframing thoughts constructively after setbacks prevents downward spirals. Acceptance and self-compassion during suffering can ameliorate emotional pain. Spiritual practices provide comfort for some. Key is tailoring constructive strategies to each life phase as needs evolve. Emotional resilience depends on honoring our changing requirements across the lifespan.

Activities That Enhance Emotional Wellbeing
Creative arts like writing, music, drama and visual arts allow healthy processing and sharing of emotions. Playing with children and pets lifts mood through joy and oxytocin release. Humor provides powerful stress relief by shifting perspective. Spiritual practices meaningfully unite communities and provide comfort through rituals and inspiration. Service to others needing help counters depression stemming from self-focus. Being in nature soothes the mind while increasing awe and gratitude. Exercise benefits both body and mind. Relaxing activities like yoga, massage and mindfulness meditation reduce anxiety. Talk therapy facilitates airing fears and gaining support. Cognitive Behavioral Therapy reframes distorted thinking patterns. Support groups aid in not feeling alone during difficult times. Antidepressant medications can help rebalance biochemistry during acute distress under medical supervision. A multifaceted approach across the lifespan boosts emotional fitness.

Strengthening Mental Health Through Lifestyle Factors
Lifestyle habits significantly impact emotional resilience. Good sleep quality and duration boosts mood and fortifies against stress. Nutritious anti-inflammatory diets increase neurotransmitter synthesis while lowering inflammation underlying mood disorders. Avoiding recreational drugs, excessive alcohol and stimulants prevents destabilizing neurochemistry. Engaging work, passions and purposeful hobbies strengthen fulfillment. Nourishing relationships provide meaning, modeling and accountability. Physical activity releases feel-good endorphins and stress-reducing norepinephrine. Finding positive mentors prevents rejection sensitivity and despair. Managing illnesses and medications that affect emotions may require professional support. Travel and new experiences counteract stagnation. Continued growth and contribution combat purposelessness. Protecting time for

renewal activities like music, reading or gardening ensures emotional nourishment. When lifestyle nurtures mental health, challenges feel surmountable.

Inspiring Examples of Emotional Resilience
Many high achievers overcame major adversities through emotional resilience. Examples include: Abraham Lincoln battling depression to lead America through its darkest chapter; Helen Keller living a stimulating life though blind and deaf; Viktor Frankl surviving Holocaust concentration camps by finding meaning through suffering; Malala Yousafzai continuing education activism after being shot for advocating for girls' schooling; Michael J.Fox tirelessly working on Parkinson's research though suffering from it; Magic Johnson combating HIV stigma through education and sports business success; Marie Curie pioneering radioactivity science as a female in a male-dominated field; Tyler Perry succeeding in media despite an abusive childhood; Oprah Winfrey overcoming trauma to inspire and connect millions; J.K. Rowling endured depression, bankruptcy and loss before Harry Potter success; Nelson Mandela forgave decades of unjust imprisonment to unify and heal. Emotional agility enables transcending pain to thrive.

Conclusion
Our emotional lives develop gradually as we build coping skills through experiencing joys and sorrows. Adversity will naturally arise but we can prepare by strengthening social support networks and therapeutic outlets. Setting developmentally appropriate challenges to achieve mastery fosters confidence. Self-awareness and self-care practices enable regulating emotions constructively. Staying actively engaged socially, intellectually and physically provides needed balance. Seeking meaning, creativity and humor sustains us through loss. No life stage is immune to suffering - childhood launches our emotional patterns while aging brings reflection and letting go.

However, at any age emotional resilience can be cultivated by honoring our evolving needs, nurturing our mental health through lifestyle, and believing in our ability to constructively adapt. With compassion, courage and wisdom accrued from life's diverse experiences, we become more agile at managing both positive and negative emotions. Our emotional lives enrich our shared human experience.

Chapter 4
Discovering Meaning and Purpose at Any Age

A sense of meaning and purpose provides satisfaction and enhances wellbeing. Purpose gives direction through pursuing goals aligned with values, belonging to communities, and contributing daily through roles. Meaning stems from transcendence, spirituality, creativity, and relationships. This chapter explores discovering purpose and meaning across life phases.

Childhood

Nurture children's innate curiosity and interests to uncover their talents and sparks. Expose them to diverse activities, hobbies, and subjects. Help them join groups and teams based on shared interests. Collaborate on family projects teaching teamwork. Discuss potential careers connected to their strengths. Recognize their accomplishments. Enable them to experiment with different identities before solidifying. Building diverse friendships expands perspectives. Allow freedom to learn from mistakes in a safe environment. Help them find meaning in learning, creation and Play.

Adolescence

Guide teens in exploring subjects and extracurricular activities they feel passionate about. Help them identify their core values and abilities to inform future educational and career paths. Discuss ways to contribute through volunteering that resonates with them. Encourage developing their belief systems and finding spiritual meaning if desired. Support relationships and creative outlets that provide a sense of belonging. Emphasize their inherent value versus tying worth to achievements. Help them balance short-term fun with long-term purpose. Foster emotional intelligence and resilience to handle setbacks. Enable them to find meaning in their interests, connections and growth journey.

Early Adulthood

Mentor young adults on finding intrinsically motivating work aligned with their strengths if possible. Discuss volunteering alongside careers to give back. Encourage cultivating relationships and community belonging through sports teams, religious groups, networking associations etc. Support creativity, learning and travel pursuits that provide enrichment. Urge broadening perspectives by engaging with different cultures. Emphasize life balance, self-care and managing stress to avoid burnout. Help them define personal values to guide decisions. Share wisdom from your own purposeful living while letting them find their own way. Help them align daily choices with long-term meaning.

Midlife

Reflect deeply on what aspects of your work and life bring the most joy, meaning and fulfillment. Make purposeful choices guided by your values, not just obligations. Reignite latent passions through hobbies, clubs or classes. Consider career mentoring to share your purpose with younger professionals. Reassess priorities and activities that drain versus uplift you. Spend time in nature to rediscover wonder and meaning. Deepen spiritual practices that provide comfort. Strengthen relationships that matter most. Express gratitude by thanking those who shaped you. Keep growing through self-improvement goals and new experiences. Leave a meaningful legacy for the next generation.

Later Life

Retirement provides opportunities to rediscover purpose. Explore enriching classes, instructing others, mentoring youth, writing memoirs, or volunteering with organizations you care about. Travel meaningfully to learn about different cultures. Share your wisdom and life lessons to support family members. Participate in religious community services that provide comfort. Spend time immersed in nature's beauty and contemplation. Discover new purposes like cooking, gardening, arts or volunteering. Reflect on how to leave a positive legacy. Derive meaning from relationships with grandchildren, friends and spiritual community members. Express gratitude for each day. Find purpose in intellectual growth, creativity and daily accomplishments however small.

Conclusion

The human need for meaning and purpose persists across life but evolves based on changing priorities and roles at each phase. Childhood is about pursuing interests, making contributions at home and school, and exploring identities. Adolescence and young adulthood focus on values development, relationships, education and career. Midlife requires reassessing meaning given new responsibilities and goals. Retirement enables discovering new purposes and leaving legacies. At any age, aligning activities with values, helping others, learning continuously, connecting authentically, finding transcendence and expressing creativity breeds meaning. By living intentionally, we uncover our unique purpose and possibilities for growth at every age. The pursuit of purpose enriches life's journey.

Chapter 5

Cultivating Strong Social Connections For Health And Happiness Across Life

Human beings are inherently social creatures, wired for connection. Extensive research conclusively demonstrates that close, supportive relationships are vital for both physical and emotional health across the human lifespan. Caring friendships, intimate romantic partnerships, and bonded familial relationships provide meaning and purpose, reduce stress and depression, increase self-worth and deliver life satisfaction. This chapter explores evidence-based strategies for developing and maintaining strong, positive social connections from childhood through adulthood and older age. Social connection is a fundamental human need on par with needs for food and shelter. By prioritizing relationships and thoughtfully nurturing our bonds with others, we can enhance our wellbeing and build lives rich in meaning, mutual support and shared memories.

Childhood

Give infants ample affection, facial engagement, responsiveness and encouragement of their babbles and curiosities to build secure attachment, trust and confidence. Hold, rock, sing lullabies, read books aloud, play finger games, and chat about their world - all nurturing cognitive and emotional development. Monitor toddlers' early friendships on playgrounds and in playgroups. Kindly coach sharing toys, taking turns, resolving conflicts and being considerate. Celebrate their budding independence while still providing a secure base. Foster preschoolers' talents and interests to grow self-esteem. Transport them to social activities like sports teams, dance classes or martial arts to widen supportive peer connections. Schedule play dates rotating between different children's homes to deepen social bonds. Meet their friends' parents to ensure positive mutual influences. Model healthy relationship behaviors through your own conduct with loved ones. Teach children forgiveness, empathy and gratitude through caring actions big and small, community service and modeling inclusive behaviors. Eat family meals together to enable relaxed bonding and conversation. Set aside one-on-one time with each child reading, playing, or discussing their interests. Provide reassurance when needed. Guide them through emotional upsets with validation, calming routines and compromise solutions. Show unconditional devotion, even when disciplining, to build secure attachment across the developmental years.

Adolescence

Respect expanding autonomy needs while remaining involved, interested and supportive as teens navigate intense social challenges and opportunities. Get to know their friends to influence positive selection and monitor for negative peer pressure. Meet other parents to kindly address any concerning behaviors together versus singularly blaming. Discuss characteristics of healthy romantic relationships, warning signs of dating abuse and the importance of consent. Talk through appropriate digital etiquette, cautions about social media oversharing and crafting online personas. Urge balance between online and in-person interactions. Remain vigilant about potential bullying or exclusion both online and in real world settings. Maintain trusted communication channels for teens to discuss relationships, sexuality, substance use, mental health or other sensitive topics without judgment. Acknowledge and validate their turbulent emotions around identity formation, social anxiety and sensitivity to rejection. Model calm, fair conflict resolution and perspective taking during family disagreements. Make home a stable, relaxed refuge for teens and their friends to congregate comfortably. Involve teens in planning family activities and traditions that preserve needed togetherness amid growing independence. Allow increasing autonomy appropriate to demonstrated maturity level. Keep the doors open but avoid invasive hovering.

Young Adulthood

Foster continual connection and support as young adults move away for college or career beginnings, establishing their new worlds apart from the daily family unit. Continue to provide practical guidance when sought without excessive unsolicited advice. Offer praise for responsibility and self-sufficiency shown. Express curiosity and interest in their studies, jobs, new friends and communities versus only conveying hurt over decreased closeness. Be enthusiastic when introduced to significant others and include them in family events when comfortable. Share positive memories that reinforce family identity and demonstrate your unconditional support and pride. Stay involved through visits, introducing them to contacts that may be helpful, and sending supportive notes or care packages during stressful periods like exam weeks or job searches. Remain home base - welcoming their friends, providing meals, laundry and moral support during return visits. Communicate using their preferred methods like texting or social media sharing while still sending old-fashioned letters or postcards too. Celebrate holidays and milestones together, adapting to shifting dynamics like including serious partners. Let go with love, allowing them to make their own choices while still imparting hard-earned wisdom when sought. Your relationship will evolve but remain vitally important through ongoing expressions of support.

Midlife

Actively strengthen marital friendship through weekly date nights - just the two of you enjoying dinner out, seeing movies, trying new activities. Get away on weekend trips sans kids whenever possible. Set aside relaxed couple time checking in daily without distractions. Discuss problems objectively when they arise, and with calm, loving communication focused on resolution versus blame. Commit to openness, forgiveness, humor, intimacy and adapting to change together as lifelong partners. Amid busy midlife responsibilities, schedule regular one-on-one time with each child, whether teen or adult. Stay attuned to their evolving needs and perspectives. Offer specific guidance on navigating relationships, education, careers and life skills only when sought. Validate their emotions. Provide practical and emotional support with grandchildren if requested. Show interest in expanded family like sons/daughters-in-law. Socialize regularly with friends through book clubs, sports teams, mom groups and couple's nights out. Share meaningful conversations not just superficial talk. Get involved in community, religious or interest groups to widen your social circle. Set boundaries with toxic people who leave you feeling depleted but keep building new connections, never taking loved ones for granted. Check in regularly on aging parents and in-laws, helping them maintain social activities too. Show daily appreciation to long-time friends and family through shared jokes and memories that reinforce bonds. Thoughtfully invest in the relationships that matter most.

Later Life
Spend meaningful time with family reminiscing over cherished memories and capturing new ones together through photos, videos, scrapbooks and shared projects like cooking traditional recipes. Regularly communicate love, pride and sincere interest in their lives through calls, letters, texts, social media and visits. Offer compliments and praise. Attend grandchildren's events, milestones and activities when possible. Share wisdom and lessons learned from your life experiences. Contribute practically through childcare, financial help with tuition, down payments or mentoring if you are able and they are receptive. Respect generational boundaries when offering advice - listen more than lecturing. Cherish time spent together without making demands on their time. Remain actively engaged in long-time friendships that provide comfort and continuity. Schedule regular catch-up phone calls, coffees or potlucks if

mobility becomes limited. Also nurture new local connections to avoid isolation and depression. Join a book club, cooking class, senior center or faith community groups. Take up new hobbies like gardening, cards, or arts that connect you with like-minded peers. Share funny stories and laughter often with both family and friends. Foster intergenerational relationships through volunteering at schools, community centers or places of worship if you are able. Offer mentorship and your accumulated knowledge if appreciated. Set aside regular digital or in-person visits with supportive loved ones who uplift you emotionally and spiritually. Provide and receive care while continuing to mutually invest in relationships that give this season meaning.

Conclusion

Our social connections provide essential nourishment, meaning and support throughout each season of life's journey. While changing priorities and roles continually reshape social needs over decades, consistently applying care, empathy, vulnerability, forgiveness and time investment enables nourishing relationships from the toddler years through the sunset seasons. Our bonds reward us with friendship, purpose, self-knowledge, undying support through ups and downs, caregiving and caretaking, community and continuity between generations. Setting relationship-building as a priority in our busy lives, never taking loved ones for granted, expressing gratitude freely and generously, and engaging in small acts of service and devotion allows relationships to remain strong for many decades, even through geographic distance and evolving roles. Our social capital gives life essential flavor and underpins health and resilience. By living relationally from childhood snow forts to elder storytelling, our lives become beautifully interwoven with others into a enriching tapestry that sustains us through all seasons of life's adventure. Our connections help us weather storms and savor moments of joy.

Chapter 6

integrating optimal self-care through all life stages

Self-care refers to any activity that replenishes our mental, emotional or physical health. When wellness is made a priority, we have greater capacity to thrive in work, relationships and handle life's inevitable challenges. Optimal self-care evolves across ages and situations. This chapter offers tailored strategies for integrating self-care into daily routines at each life stage, enabling greater joy, calm and resilience. Disciplined yet balanced self-care is not selfish but rather gives us the mental space, energy and equilibrium needed to fully show up for others without depletion. By caring for our own needs, we can better care for those we love.

Young Children
Model self-care yourself through healthy eating, daily movement and honoring your need for hobbies, relaxation and socializing. Ensure children get 10-12 hours of quality, uninterrupted sleep nightly for optimal physical and mental health. Establish consistent bedtime routines. Limit digital stimulation and caffeine before bed. Provide children nutritious, balanced meals and snacks including brain-nourishing protein, produce, healthy fats and hydration. Set aside daily tranquil family downtime to connect and decompress together through reading, coloring, board games, or child-led pretend play. Take young kids outdoors to play, run freely, expend energy and explore nature daily. Allow them to unwind through creative arts, music expression and curiosity-driven activities versus structured academics only. Teach children to label and communicate their feelings and needs. Help them practice calming techniques like belly breathing, counting or visualization when upset. Avoid overscheduling extracurriculars; prioritize unstructured playtime, family rituals and one-on-one connection. Praise effort over results to build resilience. Limit excessive criticism

or comparison that damage youthful self-esteem. Model strategies for dealing with anger, sadness, anxiety or disappointment in healthy ways. Ensure regular pediatrician checkups for immunizations, growth monitoring and health guidance. Instill the foundations of lifelong wellbeing from early on.

Adolescents

Encourage teens to preserve sleep hygiene with 8-10 hours nightly for physical and mental health. Advise limiting social media, video games and phone use before bed, which disrupt sleep. Keep a nourishing supply of healthy snacks available to avoid poor diet and recognition that hunger impacts mood. Caution teens about destructive self-care habits like substance use, eating disorders, cutting and risky sexual behaviors some teens adopt to cope with stress, anxiety or depression. Suggest journaling about feelings, playing music, drawing, painting or meditating to process emotions in a healthy way instead. Check in on their mental health regularly and watch for signs of depression, addiction or self-harm, getting professional help if needed. Model self-care yourself through healthy lifestyle habits, stress management strategies, boundary setting and honoring your own need for hobbies, exercise and socializing. Make your home a completely judgement-free zone for teens to openly discuss their feelings and struggles without fear of criticism. Teach techniques like timeouts, brisk walking, boxing, deep breathing exercises or short guided meditations to manage anxiety, anger or disappointment constructively. Help teens set priorities in academics, activities and part-time jobs so obligations don't overwhelm needed downtime. Ensure regular medical checkups and access to counseling if desired. Supportive social connections boost teenage self-worth so facilitate these.

Young Adults

Advise young adults to take full vacation time and frequent mental health days off from demanding jobs to prevent burnout. Discourage over-reliance on unhealthy coping mechanisms like alcohol, drugs, self-isolation or venting anger. Build stress-relieving recreational activities into most days, even in small ways, such as team sports, solo exercise like running, yoga classes or time in nature for mental health protection. Make relaxation practices like meditation, massage, mindfulness and counseling regular lifelong habits versus occasional emergency interventions. Model and encourage strong work-life balance through enforcing boundaries around working hours, not checking emails constantly, and honoring days off and vacation time. Nurture close family ties and friendships that provide support, perspective and care. Create nourishing morning and bedtime rituals like journaling gratitude, prayer, reflection or drinking calming tea. Prioritize 8 full hours of quality sleep nightly. Use weekends for preferred rejuvenating activities, not just chores and errands. Set clear boundaries with colleagues, clients and bosses around limited contact during personal time. Don't neglect emotional self-care through counseling, art therapy, spirituality or support groups. Stay intimately connected to uplifting family and friends who replenish you. Ignoring self-care leads to poor mental, physical and relationship health.

Midlife

Commit to prioritizing self-care amidst demanding midlife responsibilities. Maintain hobbies like gardening, golf, painting or reading novels that rejuvenate you and that you schedule time for weekly. Get away regularly for girlfriend weekends and date nights with your partner for fun, connection and romance. Exercise most days of the week, even if just a daily 20-30 minute morning energizing walk or home yoga video. Prepare healthy snacks and meals over the weekends using meal delivery kits/services to avoid daily fast food and burnout. Limit caffeine, sugar and alcohol, which disrupt sleep. Wind down screens an hour before bed. Go to bed 30 minutes earlier to ensure 7-8 hours of quality sleep nightly. Upon waking, take just 10 minutes for meditation, prayer, stretching, journaling or other ritual to start the day peacefully. At work, stand up, stretch and take short breaks every 1-2 hours. During lunch break, get outside for a short walk and reset. Set boundaries with colleagues and clients on limiting contact during personal time. Get professional massages, manicures or other self-care treats monthly. Consider counseling or support groups to healthily process work, marriage, parenting or caregiving strains before they become overwhelming. Practice saying no to nonessential obligations. Don't completely abandon hobbies, socializing and vacations that brighten your life. Ask family to support your needs too.

Later Life

Retirement provides long-awaited opportunities to refocus on consistent self-care and do activities purely for your enjoyment. Create a daily routine incorporating the self-care practices that best support your wellbeing. Enjoy leisurely mornings free of obligations with time to read books, listen to uplifting music, journal or sip tea before starting your day. Socialize frequently with friends over leisurely coffees, potlucks, matinees or museums. Join clubs for hobbies like gardening, cards or books that provide joy and social connections. Take relaxing baths or naps on your own schedule. Hand over strenuous household chores to others if needed. Stay active with preferred exercise like senior swims, walks or stretching classes tailored to your abilities and energy level. Meditate, pray or enjoy quiet contemplation. Write your memoirs or poetry. Stay meaningfully engaged in family lives through visits, calls and outings together. Protect ample time to relax and do exactly as you please without guilt. Eliminate stressful relationships from your life. Focus on nurturing mind, body and spirit daily. Light candles, play beautiful music and surround yourself with nature's beauty. Take life slowly and peacefully. Stay socially and intellectually active to avoid isolation. Honor your evolving self-care needs and limitations.

Conclusion

Wellbeing requires nurturing across our lifespans as priorities and needs evolve. The specific self-care activities we find restorative may change over the decades, but the habit of regularly caring for ourselves should remain constant. When our own needs are met, we have greater capacity to energetically care for our families, employers, friends and communities without sacrificing our health. By taking time to recharge, we can live each season of life more gracefully - reducing stress, enhancing happiness, modeling self-worth. Self-care ceases to feel self-indulgent when integrated into regular routines and instead becomes an essential practice for functioning at our best across years, relationships and occupations. Caring for yourself allows you to thrive and then thoughtfully show up for those who matter most. Make self-care a non-negotiable daily priority, not the first thing abandoned when life gets busy. Your health and community need you at your best.

Chapter 7

Adapting Lifestyles For Optimal Health And Happiness Across Life Stages

Our daily habits, routines, environments and lifestyle choices greatly impact our health, quality of life and life satisfaction across the lifespan. As we age and evolve, thoughtfully adapting our priorities, behaviors and surroundings allows us to maximize wellbeing during life's changing seasons and circumstances. This chapter explores evidence-based lifestyle adjustment strategies tailored to each stage of life, enabling us to thrive across the decades through values-based, purposeful living. With intention and willingness to make changes, we can optimize our lifestyles for fulfillment in young adulthood, midlife, older age and every phase between. By listening to our needs and crafting lifestyles aligned with our goals and abilities, we can create deeply meaningful lives from young professional to wise elder.

Young Adulthood

When gaining independence after college, beware of poor diet, erratic sleep, overwork, and social isolation. Stock your home with healthy snacks like nuts, fruits and Greek yogurt. Meal prep with friends to make cooking more social and fun. Maintain physical activity through campus recreation leagues, jogging, cycling, fitness classes or home workout apps/DVDs. Develop strong sleep hygiene, sticking to a schedule allowing 8+ hours nightly. Create an inspiring living environment with plants, natural light, cozy furniture and decor reflecting your passions. If budgets allow, choose an amenity-rich residence to reduce stress. Live within your means but allow some discretionary spending for hobbies, travel and enjoying this phase. Explore interests that energize you like hiking, dance, cultural activities or leagues. Contribute to retirement savings through work plans. Get preventative healthcare. Avoid unhealthy coping habits like heavy drinking, drugs, excessive social media or video gaming. Build lifelong positive habits now to prevent decline later. Connect to community through alumni groups, professional associations, volunteer work, sporting teams or social clubs that widen your friendships. Set ambitious yet balanced goals you feel passionate about then take purposeful, patient steps to achieve them. Find work you feel purposeful about. Develop skills continually to open new opportunities. Take risks wisely to grow confidence and resilience. Cherish family traditions and bonds amidst expanding independence.

Midlife

Adapt to evolving family needs while nurturing your marriage through weekly date nights - dinner out, shows, new hobbies together. Get away on couples' weekends when possible. Have open discussions about needs, hopes and relationship growth. Prepare healthy family meals using plans like meal prepping weekends or meal kit subscriptions. Incorporate some moderate treats. Encourage children's extracurricular activities based on their interests to discover their passions. Uphold household sleep routines for their health. Model a strong work ethic through dedication and integrity but avoid burnout through boundaries, delegating, using flextime/telework options, and taking all your vacation time. Socialize regularly with friends to maintain perspective. Stay involved in your spiritual, recreational, volunteer or special interest communities. Exercise 3-5 days a week, even if brisk morning walks or lunch break yoga sessions. Maintain leisure hobbies that refresh and fulfill you. Get preventative medical care and recommended health screenings. Continue sufficient retirement contributions. Visit aging parents often and help manage their households, finances and medical care as needed. Cherish time with family while finding purpose beyond parental roles through charitable work, professional mentoring, or special interest groups. Set meaningful new goals around personal growth, knowledge building, health metrics, career aspirations or relationship enrichment. Evaluate priorities and activities that drain versus uplift you. Protect time for self-renewal through spirituality, counseling, creativity, hobbies or escapes immersed in nature's restorative beauty. Find routines that nurture inner peace.

Later Life

Embrace a slower pace with greater flexibility in your day. Stay physically active through pool aerobics, yoga, stretching, walking or activities you most enjoy to maintain mobility, strength and pain relief. Participate in spiritually and emotionally fulfilling activities like volunteering, mentoring, teaching skills, writing, and spending quality time with family/friends. Hand over strenuous housework or yardwork to others if needed but continue doing what you can comfortably; activity promotes health. Spend time outdoors walking, gardening, appreciating nature and reminiscing. Relocate to a more convenient living space if current home maintenance becomes difficult. Consider co-housing arrangements to reduce isolation and chores while increasing affordable amenities access. Join enriching social clubs related to interests like books, travel or gardening for fun peer interactions. Take engaging community college courses to keep learning. Consider part-time work or consulting jobs that allow control over scheduling and workload. Volunteer in roles benefiting others based on your unique skills and expertise. Stay current with healthcare and get recommended senior health screens. Monitor diet, activity and medications closely. Adapt activities as needed for comfort, safety and changed abilities. Rely on your caregiving support system as needed but protect independence fiercely. Focus on each day with gratitude, optimism and active engagement versus dwelling on limitations. Protect time for tranquility in this season of life. Explore spiritual practices, mindfulness, massage and counseling for inner peace. Cherish special moments with loved ones. Reminisce by compiling photo albums, organizing long-forgotten boxes in the attic, or recording an oral history for posterity.

No matter your current life stage, strive to remain socially, intellectually and physically engaged in meaningful activities that promote health. Make regular time for vacation, hobbies, recreation, creativity and exploration to nurture your spirit. Cherish family and friends that bring you joy and purpose. Express gratitude regularly for life's blessings - a warm bed, favorite foods, children's laughter. Manage stress through self-care personalized for your needs - yoga, counseling, pets, nature walks, tea rituals. Adapt your home and daily routines to support optimal functioning as health evolves. Reduce clutter, optimize lighting, install grab bars, use rolling carts, set phone reminders. Monitor diet, sleep, activity and alcohol intake closely. Pursue purposeful goals aligned with core values versus others' expectations. Explore spirituality, meditation, art if enriching. Embrace intellectual challenge and change. Keep learning new skills to exercise your mind - take engaging courses, learn instruments, read deeply on topics of interest. Participate actively in medical decisions to manage health conditions. Focus on enjoying each day's journey while thoughtfully planning for anticipated changes ahead like moving homes, retiring, caregiving. Consider how your lifestyle may need to adapt in coming years and take proactive steps like decluttering, networking, researching options. Mindfully listen to your mind, body and spirit - they will tell you when it's time for life adjustments to honor new seasons. Trust your inner wisdom.

Conclusion

We can take control of our wellbeing at any age by thoughtfully adapting habits, surroundings and lifestyles to life's evolving seasons and our changing priorities and abilities. Each phase of life brings both gains and losses over time. With flexibility, optimism and purpose, we can maximize health and contentment throughout the decades. By listening to our needs and proactively making values-based lifestyle choices, we craft a life filled with meaning, joy and continual growth. Adapting intentionally to life's ebbs and flows allows us to blossom through all of our days. By trying new things, we keep writing new vibrant chapters. The key is maintaining curiosity, engagement and purpose year after year through conscious, responsive lifestyle design aligned with our deepest values. Life is never static - we must thoughtfully adjust and evolve as seasons change. In doing so with intention, we can create lifestyles optimized for health, purpose and passionate living during every phase - from first apartment to dream retirement. Our best life is always ahead of us if we stay open and determined.

Chapter 8

Achieving Financial Wellness to Support Health and Happiness

Achieving reasonable financial stability and security is important for reducing stress and increasing life satisfaction across the lifespan. While money alone does not guarantee happiness, having sufficient income to cover basic needs, save for goals, and provide some discretionary spending enhances peace of mind at any age. This allows us to focus energy on relationships, personal growth and enjoying life versus constantly struggling to make ends meet. This chapter offers practical financial advice tailored to each life stage for achieving financial health, the foundation that enables overall wellness. By spending mindfully, saving adequately, avoiding unnecessary debt, and investing prudently within our means, we can reduce money-related anxiety and thrive across decades.

Young Adulthood
When first living independently, create a realistic budget tracking all income and expenses using spreadsheet or budgeting apps. Pay all bills and debts on time to build strong

credit. Start saving for emergencies and establish a nest egg versus accruing credit card debt. Limit restaurant meals through cooking bulk batches of healthy meals on weekends to freeze and eat later. Look for student discounts, shop thrift stores, and buy used furnishings and essentials when possible. Learn to cut your own hair, make coffee and snacks at home, and repair your own basic electronics/appliances versus paying for services. Negotiate your best possible salary at new jobs using market data comparisons. Thoroughly understand all workplace benefits - healthcare, dental, vision, disability, life insurance, 401k plans, and other provided perks. Contribute enough to get the full employer 401k matching contribution. Explore financial assistance for further education like scholarships, grants and subsidized loans to minimize high-interest debt. If carrying existing student loans, pay the minimums while aggressively paying down highest interest loans first. Seek mentorship from financially-savvy people. Read personal finance books, blogs and take community center classes to build money management skills. Learn about investing, taxes, real estate and building wealth over decades. Live well below your means. Patience, diligence and thriftiness now lay the foundation for future comfort.

Midlife

Strive for greater income through career development, entrepreneurship or prudent investments in middle age. Actively manage childcare costs through family support systems, cost-sharing arrangements or employer benefits. Set family budgets with teens to teach financial responsibility and money habits. Make mortgage payments, life insurance and estate planning priorities before retirement. Contribute maximum amounts to tax-advantaged retirement accounts like 401ks and IRAs. Seek guidance from fee-only financial planners on investment portfolio strategies. Pay off high credit card balances and other debt draining finances using windfalls and bonuses. Reassess insurances to ensure optimal coverage for health, disability, property, auto and life based on changing needs. Specifically, increase life insurance to protect family. Aggressively save for kids' college to minimize their debt burden. Split college costs through student contributions from part-time work and careful selection of affordable in-state options. Bank any raises, bonuses or inheritances versus inflating lifestyle and spending. Communicate openly with your spouse/partner about aligning financial goals and discussing money-related stresses. Live within your total means, avoiding pressure to overspend outward displays like lavish parties or vacations. Implement smart tax filing strategies and retirement contributions to benefit your situation. Invest conservatively in a diversified, low-fee portfolio. Leave costly home renovations or luxury purchases for when better positioned. Maximize free and low-cost local entertainment and recreation with family.

Later Life

Downsize housing while home prices are favorable to fund retirement. Relocate to more affordable areas if living expenses exceed sustainable fixed income. Pay off mortgage by retirement if possible to drastically reduce expenses. At least two years before Medicare eligibility, thoroughly evaluate Parts A, B, C, D options as well as Medigap plans, factoring total costs, networks, prescription needs and risks. Sign up for Senior center memberships, AARP, and any other member discounts. Apply for any entitled pension, social security or veteran's benefits as early as age allows for maximum cumulative payments. Consult unbiased financial experts on optimizing claiming strategies and required minimum distributions from retirement accounts to minimize tax impacts. Determine essential monthly budgets as percent of fixed income for housing, food, medical, gifts/donations, discretionary and build savings for unexpected expenses. Consolidate and simply finances like rolling over 401ks and IRAs. Withdraw retirement savings judiciously at sustainable rates to avoid longevity risk. Consider annuities, longevity insurance or reverse mortgages only after thorough research and family discussion. Move assets gradually to lower-risk, income-generating investments as needed over time to preserve capital. Eliminate all consumer debt before retiring to reduce expenses. Consider continuing education or pursuing enjoyable part-time work if bored, lonely or expenses exceed projections. Live well within fixed income constraints. Enjoy travel, new adventures and making special memories with family while health permits. Gift or donate excess funds to causes important to you and leave a legacy.

Any Age

Spend mindfully and live below your income no matter what life stage. Create and stick to a realistic budget aligned with values using money management tools. Limit dining out, take-out and discretionary purchases by planning weekly menus, cooking at home, and bringing lunch to work or school. Shop sales, clip coupons, buy store brands, and frequent discount grocery and retailers. Maintain adequate emergency, retirement and education savings of at least 3-6 months' expenses. Contribute sufficient percentages of income to 401ks or IRAs up the annual maximums to accumulate enough for later years. Whenever available, fully utilize Health Savings Accounts, Flexible Spending Accounts and other tax-advantaged tools. Limit premium cable, excessive subscriptions or membership fees. Buy quality used vehicles and maintain them well while driving for many years to maximize value. Cook most meals at home and take local "staycations" versus costly vacations. Find free or low-cost recreational activities in your community using parks, trails, recreation centers and public libraries. Turn hobbies into side income through arts and crafts, mechanics skills or specialized knowledge. Use credit cards minimally, pay off monthly to avoid interest and protect scores. Automate savings for goals using payroll deductions or bank transfers. Pay all bills on time and in full to avoid penalties and interest damage. Learn DIY home/auto repairs and maintenance. Drink primarily water instead of pricier sugary beverages. Brew coffee and tea at home. Bring healthy, inexpensive lunch to work or school. Turn off lights and adjust thermostat to save energy. Research big ticket purchases thoroughly and negotiate prices for vehicles, appliances and services. Pay more upfront for durable, efficient products that save over time. Slow, steady wealth-building lasts. Patience and perseverance are key.

Conclusion

Achieving financial stability and security at any age involves spending mindfully, saving adequately, avoiding unnecessary debt, and investing wisely within your means. While specific priorities evolve across life stages, consistently living below your income, maintaining sufficient savings, and making prudent financial choices enables worry-free retirement and freedom to enjoy life's journey. With diligent budgeting, smart money habits and informed financial decisions, we can develop enough wealth to live comfortably, pursue interests, help family, gift charities, and leave a meaningful legacy without fear of scarcity. By treating finances as a key component of overall wellness, we can protect ourselves from money-related stress. Financial peace ultimately enables thriving across decades by removing the distractions of material constraints. With basic needs covered, we can focus energy on faith, family, purposeful work, travel adventures and new beginnings knowing a safety net exists thanks to our mindful financial stewardship. Wise money management allows fully engaging in life's possibilities decade after decade.

Conclusion

Living Intentionally for Health and Happiness Across Your Lifespan

Through our exploration in these chapters of evidence-based strategies for wellbeing across life seasons, some consistent themes have emerged:

Health is Holistic and Lifelong

To thrive during each life phase, we must nurture physical, mental, social, financial and spiritual health in an integrated way. This whole-person approach enables us to feel balanced and fulfilled day-to-day and pursue larger goals. For example, strong social connections improve emotional resilience which enables better stress management and cognitive performance. Exercise relieves anxiety, boosts energy for work and relationships, and lowers disease risks. Intellectual stimulation keeps the mind sharp, expands social circles, and provides purpose. Spiritual practices can enhance peacefulness, gratitude and sense of meaning. Financial diligence reduces stress while enabling better healthcare access and lifestyle options. And self-care activities like nutrition, sleep and recreation renew us to better handle life's demands. Each facet of health powerfully supports the others when developed in a holistic way over our lifespans.

Wellbeing Requires Proactivity

We must take active responsibility for bettering our health and creating lifestyles aligned with our values versus passively accepting what life hands us. This involves being proactive about medical care, self-care routines, managing stress, relationships, leisure, nature exposure, diet, fitness and financial diligence. For instance, schedule recommended health screening tests instead of only going to the doctor when sick. Dedicate consistent time for hobbies versus letting them fall by the wayside when busy. Invest upfront in relationships through shared activities rather than losing touch over the years. Plan regular vacations and time in nature that recharge you instead of endless work obligations. Prepare healthy meals rather than grabbing takeout after a tiring day. Set automatic retirement contributions versus hoping to save later. A passive approach fails us, especially as we encounter new challenges in midlife and later years. We must listen to our evolving needs across life seasons and thoughtfully respond through priorities and lifestyle design optimized for each phase.

Growth Mindset Underpins Resilience

Viewing life as an ongoing journey of learning and betterment promotes resilience in facing adversities and change. This growth mindset emerges from emotional intelligence, flexibility, curiosity to try new things, and ability to reframe struggles as temporary setbacks or learning curves rather than personal failures. For example, a job loss or accident can be seen as a pivot point to new opportunities versus the end of a plan. Chronic illness may spur developing greater patience, wisdom and appreciation for interdependence. Aging can be embraced as gaining the gifts of experience, perspective and time freedom. Believing our best chapters lie ahead galvanizes us to persevere and continue thriving through all life stages with this forward-looking mindset. Combine realistic assessment of changing capabilities with optimism and an adaptive attitude. Each phase of life offers chances for our next chapter of growth.

Prioritizing Wellbeing Enables Thriving

Taking time consistently for self-care, close relationships, recreation, nature, spirituality and other wellbeing essentials provides energy that allows us to then productively focus at work, support our families, and make a difference in our communities. Our health enables us to show up fully for others without burning out. By caring for ourselves first, we expand our capacity for thriving and serving in all of life's roles. For instance, taking a lunchtime nature walk clears our mind for afternoon productivity. An evening bath or reading relaxes so we engage warmly with loved ones later. Regular massages ease accumulated tensions enhancing calmness and patience. Adequate sleep allows having the focus to care for a sick child during the night if needed. Date nights strengthen partnerships to model a loving family. Planning budgets ensures we can generously support causes. When wellbeing is nurtured through consistent attention to mind, body and soul, our actions become powered by renewed motivation, wisdom and compassion.

Purpose and Passion Sustain Us
Pursuing purpose and meaning through family, volunteering, creativity and using our talents keeps us positively engaged across decades. Passions energize us even amidst adversity. For example, an artist keeps creating despite old age, chronic pain or shifting abilities. A teacher transforms young lives despite low pay and challenges. New parents thrive on caretaking despite sleeplessness. A devoted son visits his ailing mother daily. Volunteering at the food bank provides meaning after retirement from a dissatisfying career. Building something with your hands - whether a quilt or woodworking project - connects you to generations of skilled craftsmen before, leaving a legacy. Seeking wisdom, intellectual growth and sharing knowledge uplift our later years. Living by our values and shaping legacy infuses daily living with profound satisfaction. Purpose is found not in future circumstances but how we approach each moment and contribution.

Financial Security Enables Choices
Achieving reasonable financial stability and freedom enhances wellbeing by enabling more life options - education, career and location changes, healthcare choices, and retirement flexibility. For example, wise saving early on allows downsizing houses while prices are favorable. Investing in 401ks helps maintain lifestyle in later years. Avoiding excessive college debt burden

allows switching careers. Low-cost community college classes enable intellectual engagement post-retirement. Owning long-term care insurance affords quality choices. Not fearing basic needs allows sabbaticals, volunteering and family time. Shared budgeting and financial mentoring of youth prevents mistakes. While money itself does not drive happiness, prudent financial stewardship reduces stress throughout decades while expanding important life choices when values align with spending.

Adaptability Allows Growth

Life brings both gains and losses over time. By adapting thoughtfully to evolving capabilities, priorities and responsibilities as we age, we continue maturing through life's changing seasons. For example, a busy CEO prepares for retirement by adding volunteering to begin a different kind of meaningful contribution. A widower stays socially engaged through senior center activities versus isolation. Physical decline from arthritis is met with using canes, handrails and participating in water exercises. Loss of parents who once provided childcare leads to forming cooperative babysitting exchanges with other parents. Relocation to warmer climates when shoveling snow becomes difficult. While such adaptations require flexibility and mourning what we leave behind, we continue finding fulfillment in each life phase when we adjust thoughtfully. The key is maintaining curiosity, purpose and willingness to learn as we encounter new seasons. An adaptive attitude enables personal growth for decades to come.

Conclusion

Our daily lifestyle choices and habits at any age allow us to craft lives of purpose, wisdom, generosity and vibrancy for decades to come. While each phase of life has unique needs, an integrated focus on whole person wellbeing sustains health and happiness across the lifespan. Physical vitality gives us energy to fully participate. Emotional resilience provides tools to adapt and reframe challenges. Mental sharpness allows us to keep learning and contributing our knowledge and talents. Quality relationships deliver joy while giving meaning and support through ups and downs. Discovering passions and purpose propels us forward. Adjusting environments and routines allows maintaining engagement. Financial diligence grants peace and opportunities. By applying evidence-based wellbeing strategies tailored to our evolving needs across the years, we create deeply fulfilling legacies through all of life's seasons from childhood to the sunset seasons. May the insights gleaned serve you well on your life adventure!

www.ingramcontent.com/pod-product-compliance
Lightning Source LLC
Chambersburg PA
CBHW071033260726
48661CB00007B/3017